The Ultimate Diet Cookbook
BOX- SET 2 IN 1:

25 Tasty Recipes Will Help You To Lose
Weight Fast & Easy + Lose 10 Lbs In 10
Days! 20 Delicious Ketogenic Recipes For
Healthy Weight Loss

Table of contents

Book 1

Book 2

LOW CARB DIET PLAN

NADENE SMITH

25 TASTY RECIPES

Will Help You To Lose Weight Fast & Easy!

Low Carb Diet Plan

25 Tasty Recipes That Will Help You Lose Weight Fast & Easy!

Introduction

Low carbohydrate diets aim to limit your daily carbohydrate intake, such as carbohydrates that are found in starchy vegetables, fruits, and grains. These types of diets also emphasize eating more fat and protein to make up for cutting back on the carbohydrates. Every diet is different, and every low carbohydrate diet is different on the amount of carbohydrates that are limited. In this book, you're going to find low carbohydrate recipes that are generally safe for all low carbohydrate diets.

Many people try low carbohydrate diets to lose weight, but there are more benefits to these types of diets than just weight loss. Low-carbohydrate diets will reduce your risk factors associated with metabolic syndrome and diabetes. They're also excellent for those who are looking for a more heart healthy lifestyle.

Carbohydrates form naturally in plant-based foods like grains. In their natural state, they can be complex and take longer to digest, like the carbohydrates found in legumes and whole grains, or they can be less complex, like the ones found in fruit and milk. Some common sources of all types of carbohydrates include fruits, grains, milk, vegetables, seeds, nuts, and legumes.

However, in addition to there being natural carbohydrates, there are also the ones that are added to processed foods. The two most common refined carbohydrates added to processed foods are sugar and flour. They're known as simple carbohydrates because the body is able to process them with a lot less energy and fewer steps to getting them converted into fat. Examples of foods that contain these types of carbohydrates include cake, cookies, pasta, sugary sodas and fruit drinks, and candy.

The body uses carbohydrates, both simple and complex, in order to keep working. Starches and sugars get broken down into simple sugars through the process of digestions, and then are absorbed into the bloodstream. They're known as glucose then. Carbohydrates that contain fiber will resist digestion and have a lower effect ton blood sugar. They also provide bulk and will provide other bodily functions with fuel, too.

Carbohydrates help your body by raising the levels of blood sugar, which will raise the levels of insulin in the body. Insulin then helps the glucose enter the body's cells, and some of that glucose is used for energy while extra glucose is then stored in muscles, the liver, or as fat. The idea behind a low carbohydrate diet is to decrease the carbohydrates in order to lower the insulin levels, which then encourage the body to burn stored fat rather than extra glucose entering the bloodstream. This ultimately will lead to weight loss.

So what foods are common in a low carbohydrate diet? Most low-carbohydrate diets put an emphasis on consuming a lot of protein, so poultry, red meat, eggs, and fish are considered safe.

In addition, non-starchy vegetables are also considered conducive to weight loss. Foods to avoid would include pasta, sweets, legumes, fruits, bread, starchy vegetables, and sometimes seeds and nuts. However, all low carbohydrate diets are different, and some will allow pasta and bread as long as they are truly whole grain, and fruit, too.

Most low-carbohydrate diets will limit the carbohydrate intake to sixty to a hundred and thirty grams of carbs per day. They will provide around two hundred and forty to five hundred and twenty calories per day. Therefore, the recipes in this book will focus on a goal of between sixty and a hundred and thirty grams of carbs per day.

So if you're ready to get started on your weight loss journey with some delicious recipes, then keep reading!

Chapter 1 – Breakfast Recipes for Champions

Breakfast is a very important part of your day because what you choose to eat for breakfast will influence what you choose to eat for lunch, dinner, and snacks. So choose one of these healthy, delicious breakfasts to jumpstart your day!

Baked Eggs with Spinach, Yogurt, and Chili Oil

Servings: 2-4

Carbohydrates per Serving: 19.6g

Ingredients

2/3 C. Plain Greek Yogurt

1 Clove Garlic, Halved

Pinch of Salt

2 Tbsp. Unsalted Butter, Divided

2 Tbsp. Olive Oil

3 Tbsp. Chopped Leek

2 Tbsp. Chopped Scallion

10 C. Spinach (10 Oz.)

1 Tsp. Lemon Juice

4 Eggs

1/4 Tsp. Turkish Chili Powder

1 Tsp. Chopped Oregano

Directions

1. Combine the yogurt through the salt in a bowl and allow to rest.

2. Preheat your oven to 300 degrees Fahrenheit and melt a tablespoon of butter with the oil in a cast-iron skillet. Sauté the leek and scallion until they're soft, around ten minutes. Add the spinach and the lemon juice, season with a little salt, and increase the heat to medium-high. Cook four to five minutes, turning until it's wilted.

3. Place the spinach in a ten-inch skillet and leave the excess liquid in the pan. Make four indentations in the center of the skillet with the spinach and break one egg into the indentations. Bake the skillet until the egg whites are cooked, around fifteen minutes.

4. Melt a tablespoon of butter in a saucepan over some medium heat and add the Turkish chili powder with a little salt. Cook around two minutes. Then add the oregano and cook another thirty seconds.

5. Remove the garlic from the yogurt and spoon it over the spinach and eggs. Drizzle with the butter sauce.

Chocolate Hazelnut Granola

Servings: 10

Carbohydrates per Serving: 9.8g

Ingredients

1 + 1/2 C. Hazelnuts

1 + 1/2 C. Almonds

1 C. Flax Seed Meal

1/4 C. Cocoa Powder

1/2 Tsp. Salt

1/4 C. Butter, Melted

1/4 C. Hazelnut Oil

2 Oz. Unsweetened Chocolate

1/3 C. Sweetener

1/2 Tsp. Hazelnut Extract

20 Drops Stevia Extract

Directions

1. Preheat your oven to 300 degrees Fahrenheit and line a baking sheet with some parchment paper.

2. Process the hazelnuts and almonds in a food processor until they look like breadcrumbs with a few large pieces. Place in a bowl and stir in the flax seed meal through the salt.

3. In a saucepan, heat the butter, oil, and chocolate over low heat until it's smooth. Stir in the sweetener.

4. Remove the pan from the heat and stir in the extracts.

1. Pour the chocolate over the nut mix and toss it to combine. Allow some to clump together.

2. Spread on the baking sheet and bake fifteen minutes, occasionally stirring, until it begins to crisp. Turn off the oven and allow the mix to sit in there another twenty minutes. Keep an eye on it so it doesn't burn.

3. Serve over yogurt or in a bowl with some unsweetened almond milk.

Blackberry Lemon Ricotta Parfaits

Servings: 6

Carbohydrates per Serving: 5.8g

Ingredients

15 Oz. Whole Milk Ricotta

3 Tbsp. Lemon Juice

2 Tsp. Lemon Zest

2 Tbsp. Powdered Sweetener

16 Drops Stevia Extract

1 C. Blackberries

1/4 C. Chopped Toasted Hazelnuts

Directions

1. Combine the ricotta through the stevia in a food processor and pulse until smooth.

2. Divide the berries amongst six cups and top with half of the ricotta mixture. Repeat with the rest of the berries and the ricotta. Sprinkle with the hazelnuts and serve.

Chapter 2 – Filling Lunch Recipes

Lunch is that time of the day where most people are willing to try something healthy. You want to eat light so you're not bogged down, but you also want to be filled up enough that you're not craving a snack mid afternoon that's of the carbohydrate-filled kind. These recipes will definitely have you feeling full but not feeling like you ate a brick, so get ready for an energy-boosting lunch!

Zesty Shrimp & Black Bean Salad

Servings: 4

Carbohydrates per Serving: 19g

Ingredients

1/4 C. Cider Vinegar

3 Tbsp. Olive Oil

1 Tbsp. Minced Chipotle Chile In Adobo

1 Tsp. Ground Cumin

1/4 Tsp. Salt

1 lb. Prepared Shrimp, Diced into 1/2" Pieces

15 oz. Can Black Beans, Rinsed

1 C. Cherry Tomatoes, Quartered

1 Poblano Pepper, Chopped

1/4 C. Scallions, Chopped

1/4 C. Cilantro, Chopped

Directions

1. Whisk together the vinegar through the salt in a bowl.

2. Add the shrimp through the cilantro and toss to coat.

3. Serve at room temperature or chill for up to three hours.

Sesame Tuna Salad

Servings: 4

Carbohydrates per Serving: 9g

Ingredients

1/4 C. Rice Vinegar

3 Tbsp. Canola Oil

2 Tbsp. Soy Sauce

1 Tbsp. Toasted Sesame Oil

1 +1/2 tsp. Sugar

1 +1/2 tsp. Minced Ginger

12 oz. Tuna Packed in Water, Drained

1 C. Sliced Sugar Snap Peas

2 Scallions, Sliced

6 C. Thinly Sliced Napa Cabbage

4 Radishes, Sliced

1/4C. Cilantro Leaves

1 Tbsp. Sesame Seeds

Salt and Pepper To Taste

Directions

1. Whisk the vinegar through the ginger in a bowl.

2. Combine three tablespoons of the dressing with the tuna through the scallions in another bowl.

3. Divide the cabbage amongst four plates and mound a fourth of the tuna mix in the center of the plates. Garnish with the radishes through the sesame seeds.

4. Drizzle with the rest of the dressing and season with salt and pepper.

Tuscan-Style Tuna Salad

Servings: 4

Carbohydrates per Serving: 20g

Ingredients

12 oz. Tuna, Drained

15 oz. Can Small White Beans, Rinsed

4 Scallions, Trimmed And Sliced

10 Cherry Tomatoes, Quartered

2 Tbsp. Olive Oil

2 Tbsp. Lemon Juice

1/4 Tsp. Salt

Salt and Pepper, To Taste

Directions

1. Combine the tuna through the salt and pepper in a bowl. Stir and refrigerate until ready to serve.

Muffin-Tin Crab Cakes

Servings: 6

Carbohydrates per Serving: 18g

Ingredients

1 lb. Crabmeat

2 C. Whole-Wheat Breadcrumbs

1/2 Red Bell Pepper, Minced

3 Scallions, Sliced

1/4 C. Mayonnaise

2 Eggs

1 Egg White

1/2 Tsp. Celery Salt

10 Dashes Hot Sauce

1/4 Tsp. Salt and Ground Pepper

6 Lemon Wedges

Directions

1. Preheat your oven to 450 degrees Fahrenheit. Coat a twelve cup muffin pan with cooking spray.

2. Mix the crab through the pepper in a bowl until combined. Divide amongst the muffin tins.

3. Bake twenty to twenty-five minutes or until crispy.

4. Serve with the lemon wedges.

Chapter 3 – Tasty Dinner Recipes

Dinner is the meal of the day where everyone gets to sit down and relax. The rough day is over and no one wants anything more than to sit around at the table with their family eating a home-cooked, comforting meal. These recipes are designed for those who are looking for something easy to prepare, as well as healthy. They're also recipes that, hopefully, the entire family will enjoy.

Tropical Fish Fillets Recipe

Servings: 4

Carbohydrates per Serving: 6g

Ingredients

4 Roughy Fillets (6 Oz. Each)

3 Tbsp. All-Purpose Flour

1 Tbsp. Butter

1/2 C. Chicken Broth

2 Tbsp. Lime Juice

1 Tbsp. Minced Cilantro

1 Tsp. Grated Lime Peel

1/2Tsp. Ground Coriander

1/4 Tsp. Ground Cumin

Directions

1. Coat the fish with the flour. In a skillet, melt the butter and place the fillets in. Cook for three minutes on either side or until the fish flakes with a fork. Remove and keep it warm.

2. In the skillet, at the rest of the ingredients and cook three minutes or until heated. Serve over the fillets.

Pork Chops with Blackberry Sauce Recipe

Servings: 4

Carbohydrates per Serving: 14g

Ingredients

4 Pork Loin Chops (7 Oz. Each)

1/4 C. Blackberry Spreadable Fruit

1/4 Tsp. Minced Garlic

3 Tbsp. Ketchup

1/4 Tsp. Prepared Mustard

1/4 Tsp. Cornstarch

1 Tbsp. Steak Sauce

Directions

1. Broil the pork chops four to five inches from the broiler for four to five minutes on either side. The thermometer should read 145 degrees Fahrenheit. Allow them to stand five minutes.

2. While the pork chops rest, combine the fruit spread through the mustard in a saucepan and bring to a boil. Combine the steak sauce with the cornstarch until it's smooth. Gradually stir it into the saucepan and bring to a boil again. Stir two minutes or until thickened.

3. Serve the pork chops with the sauce drizzled over the top.

Spinach Chicken Roll Recipe

Servings: 1

Carbohydrates per Serving: 5g

Ingredients

1 Tbsp. Onion, Chopped

1 Tsp. Olive Oil

3 C. Spinach

1/4 Tsp. Dill Weed

6 oz. Chicken Breast

2 Tbsp. Feta Cheese, Crumbled

Directions

1. In a skillet, sauté the onion in the oil until it's tender. Add the spinach and stir for two to three minutes or until it's wilted. Then stir in the dill and remove it from the heat.

2. Flatten the chicken until it's around a quarter inch thick and place the spinach and feta cheese along the center. Fold a side over the filling and roll it up tightly. Secure it with a toothpick.

3. Place it with the seam side down on the skillet and cook for fifteen to twenty minutes, covered.

Mushroom Beef Stew Recipe

Servings: 9

Carbohydrates per Serving: 14g

Ingredients

32 oz. Beef Broth

1 oz. Dried Mixed Mushrooms

1/4 C. All-Purpose Flour

1 Tsp. Salt

1 Tsp. Pepper

2 lbs. Beef Chuck Roast, Cubed

3 Tbsp. Canola Oil

1 lb. Baby Portobello Mushrooms

5 Carrots, Chopped

1 Onion, Chopped

3 Clove Garlics, Minced

3 Tsp. Rosemary

2 Tbsp. Cornstarch

2 Tbsp. Cold Water

Hot Cooked Egg Noodles

1/4 C. Crumbled Blue Cheese

Directions

1. Bring the first two ingredients to a boil in a saucepan. Remove them from the heat and allow them to rest twenty minutes or until the mushrooms have become soft. Drain the mushrooms but reserve the liquid, chop the mushrooms, and set them both aside.

2. Combine the flour through the pepper in a plastic bag and set it aside. Set aside one tablespoon for the sauce. Add the beef, a couple pieces at a time, and shake it to coat.

3. Brown the beef in a Dutch oven with oil. Add the whole mushrooms through the onion and sauté until it's tender. Add the garlic with the rosemary and chopped mushrooms, cook another minute. Stir in the flour mixture until it's blended and add the mushroom broth slowly.

4. Bring to a boil and then reduce the heat. Simmer for two hours or until the beef is tender. Bring the stew to a boil, combine the cornstarch and the water until it's smooth, and stir into the pan slowly. Return it to a boil and stir two minutes or until it's thickened.

5. Serve with the egg noodles and top with the blue cheese.

6. You can also freeze this for up to six months. Thaw in the refrigerator overnight and place in a Dutch oven to reheat.

Chapter 4 – Curb Cravings with These Snacks

So you just had breakfast, lunch, or dinner and you're craving something that's going to help fill you up, but not necessarily something sweet. While there is one sweet recipe in this chapter for those who have a sweet tooth, this chapter is more about helping you feel full without loading up on carbohydrates. You can choose to serve these as snacks, sides for your main meals, or just as a late night treat. Just because you've changed your lifestyle to be healthier doesn't mean you have to starve to do it!

Cottage Cheese Veggie Dip

Servings: 1

Carbohydrates per Serving: 14g

Ingredients

1/2 C. Cottage Cheese

1/4 Tsp. Lemon Pepper

1/2 C. Baby Carrots and Snow Peas

Directions

1. Whisk together the cottage cheese and lemon pepper. Serve with the carrots and peas as a dipping sauce.

Turkey Rollups

Servings: 1

Carbohydrates per Serving: 11g

Ingredients

2 Slices Deli Turkey Breast

2 Tsp. Honey Mustard

Salt and Pepper

2 Sesame Breadsticks

Directions

1. Spread the slices of turkey with a teaspoon of mustard and season with the salt and pepper. Wrap them around one breadstick.

Edamame Nibbles

Servings: 16

Carbohydrates per Serving: 5g

Ingredients

4 C. Frozen Edamame, Cooked

2 Tsp. Coarse Salt

Directions

1. Toss the cooked edamame with the salt and enjoy!

Five-Spice Pistachios

Servings: 48 (2 Tbsps. per Serving)

Carbohydrates per Serving: 5g

Ingredients

6 Tbsp. Orange Juice

6 Tbsp. Chinese Five-Spice Powder

4 Tsp. Salt

6 C. Unsalted Pistachios

Directions

1. Preheat your oven to 250 degrees Fahrenheit with the racks in the upper and middle third of the oven.

2. Whisk the orange juice through the salt in a bowl, add the pistachios, and toss them to coat. Divide them between two baking sheets and spread into an even layer.

3. Bake them and stir every fifteen minutes for forty-five minutes or until they're dry. Let them cool on the baking sheets completely and store in an airtight container.

Chapter 5 – Late Night Dessert Recipes

It's the chapter you've been hoping to find! Yes, you get to have dessert when you're on a low-carbohydrate diet. You just have to be a little sparing with it and you get to use some ingredients you may not have found at your local grocery store. Try looking in the organic aisle or looking at a local health food market for some of the ingredients found in these recipes. You won't regret you spent the extra time!

Go ahead, enjoy dessert!

Lemon Squares

Servings: 18

Carbohydrates per Serving: 2.4

Ingredients

1 C. Almond Flour

1/4 Tsp. Sea Salt

2 Tbsp. Sugar Substitute

1 Tbsp. Coconut Oil, Melted

2 Tbsp. Unsalted Butter, Melted

1 Tbsp. Vanilla Extract

1/4 C. Almond Flour

1/4 C. Sugar Substitute

2 Tsp. Stevia

4 Eggs

1/2 C. Squeezed Lemon Juice

Directions

1. Preheat your oven to 350 degrees Fahrenheit and line an eight-inch baking dish with parchment paper.

2. Combine the almond flour through the sea salt in a bowl. In another bowl, stir together the coconut oil through the vanilla extract. Stir the wet into the dry ingredients until it's combined. Press the dough into the prepared baking dish. Bake seventeen minutes.

3. While the crust is baking, start the topping. In a blender, pulse the almond flour through the lemon juice together. Remove the crust from the oven and pour the topping over the hot crust.

4. Place back in the oven and bake another twenty minutes at 350 degrees Fahrenheit. The topping should be golden around the edges. Allow it to cool for thirty minutes in the baking dish and refrigerate for two hours to set. Sprinkle with the powdered sugar and cut into bars and serve.

Chocolate-Dipped Apricots

Servings: 36

Carbohydrates per Serving: 4g

Ingredients

1/2 C. Bittersweet Chocolate Chips

36 Dried Apricots

2 Tbsp. Chopped Pistachios

Directions

1. Line your baking sheet with some wax or parchment paper.

2. Place the chocolate chips in a glass bowl that's safe for the microwave. Microwave on medium for a minute. Stir, and continue microwaving at twenty-second intervals until it's melted.

3. Dip half an apricot into the melted chocolate and allow the excess chocolate to drip back into the bowl. Place the fruit on the prepared baking sheet and sprinkle with the pistachios.

4. Refrigerate thirty minutes or until the chocolate is set.

Apple Zucchini Crisp

Servings: 9

Carbohydrates per Serving: 10g

Ingredients

1 C. Apples, Peeled And Thinly Sliced

2 C. Zucchini, Peeled, Halved And Thinly Sliced

1/4 C. Splenda Brown Sugar

2 Tsp. Cinnamon, Divided

A Pinch Of Nutmeg

3 Tbsp. Lemon Juice

1/3 C. Almond Meal

1/3 C. Sliced Almonds

1/3 C. Chopped Pecans

1 Tsp. Vanilla Extract

1/4 C. Butter, Melted

Directions

1. Preheat your oven to 375 degrees Fahrenheit.

2. Toss the apples through the lemon juice and a teaspoon of cinnamon in a bowl together.

3. Pour them into an eight by eight baking dish.

4. Mix the brown sugar with the last teaspoon of cinnamon through the pecans together in a separate bowl.

5. Stir the vanilla and melted butter into the nut mixture and mix well.

6. Crumble the nut mix over the apples and zucchini.

7. Bake for thirty minutes uncovered.

8. Top with some whipped cream.

Cinnamon-Sugar Cookies

Servings: 25

Carbohydrates per Serving: 7g

Ingredients

1 +1/2 C. All-Purpose Flour

1 +1/2 C. Whole-Wheat Flour

1/4 Tsp. Baking Soda

1/4 Tsp. Salt

1 +1/4 Tsp. Baking Powder

3 Tsp. Ground Cinnamon, Divided

1 C. Plus 1 Tsp. Sugar, Divided

4 Tbsp. Unsalted Butter

5 Tbsp. Canola Oil

2 Tsp. Vanilla Extract

2 Eggs

Directions

1. You can store the wrapped rolls of dough in the freezer for up to three months and make cookies when you desire.

2. Whisk the white whole-wheat flour with the all-purpose flour and two teaspoons of cinnamon, the baking powder, baking soda, and salt in a bowl.

3. Beat a cup of sugar, oil, and butter in a mixing bowl until smooth. Add the eggs and vanilla and whisk until smooth. Add the flour mix and combine on low speed until just wet.

4. Place half the dough in plastic wrap and shape into a ten-inch log. Repeat with the rest of the dough. Freeze until firm, around forty-five minutes. Reroll them to make them rounder and return them to the freezer around one hour.

5. Preheat the oven to 350 degrees Fahrenheit and line a baking sheet with some parchment paper.

6. Remove one roll of dough from the freezer and allow it to sit at room temperature for five minutes. Unwrap and slice it into quarter into thick rounds. Place the cookies half an inch apart on the baking sheet.

7. Combine the last teaspoon of cinnamon with the sugar in a small bowl and sprinkle the cookies with a little bit.

8. Bake eight minutes and transfer to a wire rack to cool completely. Repeat with the rest of the dough.

Conclusion

As an included bonus, I'm going to give you a one day plan for your first day so that you can get started on your weight loss journey! Because most low carbohydrates like the grams of carbohydrates to be kept around sixty grams, this plan will keep it at or below sixty grams of carbohydrates on your first day. So let's get started!

Day One

Breakfast: An old-fashioned breakfast with eggs and bacon would do you well and land you in the no carbohydrates zone for breakfast, or you could get fancy and try out the Baked Eggs with Spinach, Yogurt and Chili Oil in chapter one.

Lunch: A salad with some dark, leafy greens, tomatoes, Kalamata olives, and feta cheese might land you in the 2 grams of carbohydrates area, or you could try out something more filling like the Zesty Shrimp and Black Bean Salad.

Snack: Everyone needs a snack between lunch and dinner to keep them going! On day one, try something light like some Edamame Nibbles.

Dinner: After having a day that's been successful in staying low carb, there's no point in ruining it with an unhealthy dinner. Try out the Tropical Fish Fillets Recipe.

Dessert: Who doesn't like to end the day with dessert? Try out this delicious recipe, Lemon Squares.

At the end of the day, with just one serving of every recipe, you will have consumed 52 grams of carbohydrates!

I hope you enjoyed the recipes found in this book. If so, please leave a review at your online eBook retailer's website.

Thank you for reading!

KETOGENIC
DIET COOKBOOK

Adrienne Kelly

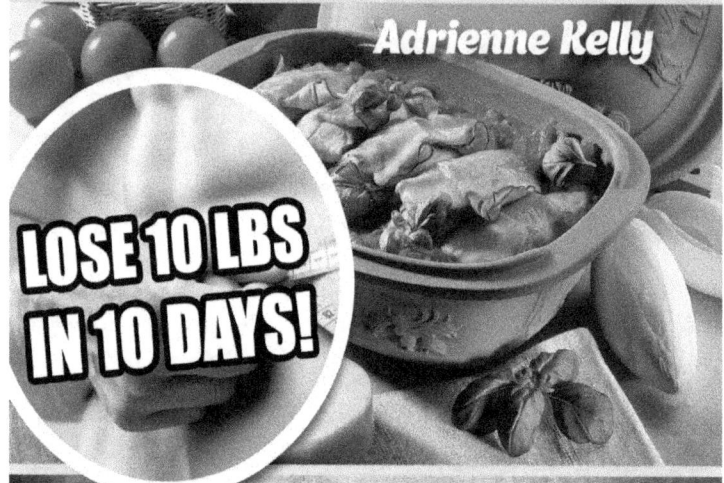

LOSE 10 LBS IN 10 DAYS!

20 *Delicious*
Ketogenic Recipes
For Healthy Weight Loss

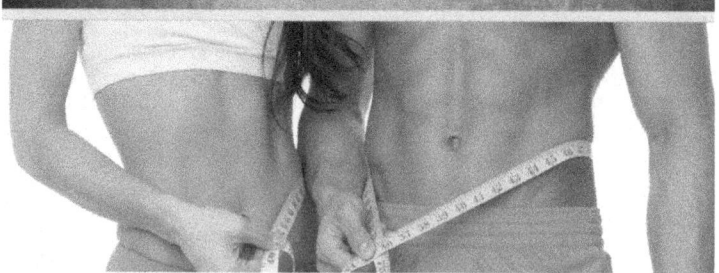

Ketogenic Diet Cookbook: Lose 10 Pounds In 10 Days!

20 Delicious Ketogenic Recipes For Healthy Weight Loss

Introduction

There you are, standing in the store again. There are so many options of what you can buy for dinner tonight, and so many things that are telling you they are the best choice for your family.

Things that claim they are baked and not fried, things that are fat free, low sodium, GMO free... you don't even know where to begin. Then you catch a glimpse of yourself in the reflection of the window, and are once again reminded of how you wish you could lose some weight, but have no idea how to begin.

That's where this book comes in. Offering recipes that will get you through your entire day, you will find that it is fast, easy, inexpensive, and convenient to use the Ketogenic diet plan to lose weight.

Using proven methods that will maximize your weight loss and give you the body you have always wanted, this cookbook will give you recipes that are not only going to help you lose weight, but are going to taste great, too.

The whole family will be more than happy to jump on board with these tasty recipes, and what makes it all even better is that you don't have to worry about breaking your budget, either, as these are all designed to taste great but be affordable for any household.

You're tired of being tired, and just want to have that body you have been dreaming of. Sometimes that feels like a lot to ask, but in reality, it's not. All you have to do is follow this simple eating plan, and use the recipes in this cookbook and you will have the body you have been craving, and not have to give up great tasting food to get it.

So what are you waiting for? Dinner is right around the corner, and so is your new jean size.

Chapter 1 – What Is the Ketogenic Diet?

The ketogenic diet is one that originated in the medical field to help people with various conditions. It works by utilizing the liver's ability to produce ketones and fatty acids that are meant to break down and use the fat in the rest of the body.

This means that by getting your liver to work with you, you will be able to break down fat and get rid of it without having to do anything but eat the delicious foods that are provided in this diet.

But what foods are those?

Quite a lot, really. The only foods that you need to avoid are those that are high in carbs. This is because carbs don't work with the liver, and, in fact, cause your body to hang onto fat rather than lose it.

So, by removing carbs from your diet and replacing them with fats and proteins, you are encouraging your liver to use these things and produce the hormones needed to get them out of your body, which, in turn, will burn off the other fat that is stored in your body as well.

But isn't there some sort of supplement that needs to help this process along?

No! The ketogenic diet is one that works with your body as it was intended to be worked with, through the food you eat. You don't have to take any supplements or worry about anything extra, just avoid carbohydrates and focus on foods like the ones we have put together in these recipes.

The only other thing you need to do is to remember to drink plenty of water. On the outset of this diet, you will lose water quickly, and that poses the risk of becoming dehydrated, but that is something that is easily avoided when you drink plenty of water all throughout your day.

Is there anything I can do that will help me retain water... besides drinking it all the time?

Salt. The answer is quite simple, and it is salt. Salt has properties to it that causes you to retain water, which is why a lot of people cut their sodium intakes. This is not what you want to do, however, if you are trying to keep water in your body.

Simply up your salt intake, which is relatively easy to do, simply add a dash of it to whatever it is you are having, and you are set. This shouldn't take the place of your water intake, but it will definitely help.

Note:

While I do encourage you to keep your water intake up, it is important that you don't drink too much water. Yes, it does take quite a bit to do this, but it is important that you are smart about this.

Drink enough water to keep yourself hydrated, but don't drink so much that it is causing problems all on its own.

The ketogenic diet really is that simple. Watch your carb intake, and your water consumption, and you are set. The pounds really will start melting off of you, and you can stick with the diet, long after your 10 days, 2 weeks, or even your month, is up.

So what's next?

Now we have reached the fun part... the recipes. These recipes all contain everything you need to be successful at this diet, and you really will see the results in a matter of days.

Feel free to adjust the amounts as needed for your own personal family size, they are all written specifically to serve 2.

Chapter 2 – Breakfast Recipes

Breakfast is by far the most important meal of the day. This is the meal that starts up your metabolism for the entire day. It is a proven fact if you skip this meal, you will not have the same level of fat burning that you do if you eat breakfast.

A lot of people skip breakfast, whether it be because they don't feel that they have enough time to eat it, or because they think they are saving on calories if they don't.

This thinking is often flawed, however, in that if you skip out on breakfast, your metabolism is unable to process the calories you put into your body the rest of the day. Another aspect is the fact that you will likely undo your hard work with lunch if you don't eat in the morning.

These recipes are all easy to make, and they are easy on the budget as well. If you are short on time, and trying to get breakfast in during a pinch, these are the meals for you.

Powerhouse Breakfast Smoothie

What you will need:

1 cup coconut milk

½ cup peanut butter

1 avocado

1 tsp vanilla

2 packets stevia

Ice

Directions:

Slice the avocado into small pieces, and toss into the blender with the rest of the ingredients, except for the ice. Place the lid on the blender and blend on medium high until all ingredients are thoroughly mixed together.

Add the ice cubes in small sections, and blend in. For a thicker smoothie, add in more peanut butter, for a thinner smoothie, add more milk.

Another benefit is that you don't taste the avocado at all, which really is a plus for those that don't like avocado.

Spicy Cheese Cakes

What you will need:

½ brick cream cheese

3 eggs

1 tablespoon almond flour

1 tsp baking powder

½ cup shredded pepper jack cheese

Salt and pepper

1 tsp vanilla

1 packet stevia

Directions:

Heat a skillet over medium high heat on the stove.

Spray with no stick spray. Soften cream cheese in microwave, until it can be mixed easily. In a mixing bowl, combine all ingredients, except pepper jack cheese.

After combined, blend in pepper jack, and, using a ladle, spoon onto skillet. Cook on each side until golden brown, about three minutes, and serve immediately.

Barnyard Omelets

What you will need:

4 eggs

½ pound breakfast sausage

A splash of milk

¼ cup bacon crumbles

1 small tomato

1 small onion

Directions:

Heat a greased skillet on the stove, and while it is preheating, beat eggs with the milk. Pour half of the eggs onto the skillet, and while it starts to brown, chop the onion and tomato.

Brown the sausage, and add half to the eggs, as well as half of the rest of the remaining ingredients.

Flip half of the omelet over, and cook until soft and firm. Repeat these steps for the second omelet. Garnish with cheese, salt, and pepper if desired.

On the Road Cereal

What you will need:

1 cup Keto cereal

½ cup dehydrated strawberries

½ cup chocolate chips

½ cup chopped almonds

¼ cup peanut butter

2 cups coconut milk

Directions:

In a mixing bowl, mix all ingredients except for the milk. Divide evenly between two serving bowls, and divide the milk between the two. Serve and enjoy immediately, as it will get soggy if it sits too long.

Broccoli Egg Bake

What you will need:

1 cup broccoli florets

¼ pound sausage

3 eggs

½ cup almond milk

1 tsp tabasco sauce

Salt and pepper to taste

Directions:

Heat a greased skillet on the stove, and chop up the florets as small as you can get them. In a mixing bowl, mix all ingredients together. Pour into the skillet, and let sit, covered, for 5 minutes.

After the eggs have sit for five minutes, transfer the whole pan into the oven preheated to 350 degrees F for 15 minutes.

Garnish with cheese and some tabasco sauce, and serve.

Chapter 3 – Lunch Recipes

Lunch is a difficult meal for many of us to squeeze into our busy days. It comes at one of the worst times in the day, and it quickly becomes way too tempting to hit the vending machine for a bag of chips rather than try to pack something healthy and eat it at work.

Lunch at work can be the hardest thing to navigate during your day. You are tired, you have been busy, and likely you are feeling hungry, especially if you didn't have breakfast that day. It is important, however, that you don't let your day come undone now, you need to stay strong and keep it together.

Your waist line will thank you, however, if you break out of this cycle and pack your own meals. They will be a lot healthier, a lot less expensive, and will help you stay on track a lot better than if you stick to what the cafeteria or vending machine have to offer.

Chicken Tomato Salad

What you will need:

2 chicken breasts

2 cups green leaf lettuce

½ cup almonds

6 grape tomatoes

Directions:

Cook the chicken breasts, and set aside. Rip up the lettuce and divide between two plates. Slice the chicken breast into strips, and lay over the lettuce. Slice the grape tomatoes into slivers, four slivers per tomato, then divide between the two plates, 12 slices per plate.

Drizzle each salad with a moderate amount of Caesar dressing, and divide the almonds between the two plates.

Serve immediately.

Garden Wraps

What you will need:

2 large lettuce leaves

1 cup lettuce (besides the leaves)

1 tomato

1 avocado

Mayo

Olives

1 small red onion

2 hardboiled eggs

Directions:

Lay out the lettuce leaves on two plates, then spread a thin layer of mayo on each leaf.

Tear up the remaining lettuce, and spread over the leaves, thinly slice the tomato and onion, and lay over the leaves as well.

Sprinkle the eggs across the leaves, and slice the avocado, then add as a final layer.

Roll the wraps around themselves, and secure with a toothpick. Serve dish immediately.

Sunrise Soup

What you will need:

4 tomatoes

1 small onion

1 cup heavy cream

1 cup coconut milk

1 summer squash

Salt and pepper

Directions:

Pour the cream and milk into a pan on the stove, and turn on low heat. As the cream is heating, chop up the tomatoes as small as you can, then do the same with the onion.

Add both of these things to the soup, and stir. Place the squash in the microwave, and cook until done. Scoop out the inside of the squash, and add to the pot on the stove.

Cook for 10 minutes, stirring often until all the ingredients are soft. Using a stick blender, blend all of the ingredients until the soup is completely smooth.

Add salt and pepper to taste, and serve.

Hamburger Hats

What you will need:

1/2 pound hamburger

4 slices bacon

2 eggs

Salt and pepper

Mayo

2 large green leaf lettuce

Tomato

Onion

Directions:

Divide the hamburger into two even sections, and form into patties. Heat a skillet on the stove, and add the bacon. Once the bacon is cooked, remove, set aside, and place the hamburger patties in the bacon grease and cook.

Add salt and pepper, and flip half way through the cooking process.

As the hamburgers are cooking, lay out the leaves on two plates, then spread two thin layers of mayo across the leaves. Slice the tomato and the onion, then remove the hamburgers from the heat.

Crack the eggs in the pan with the hamburger grease, and cook them, over easy, in the pan. As the eggs are cooking, set the hamburgers on the lettuce, then lay a slice of tomato, a slice of onion, and 2 slices of bacon per hamburger.

Season the eggs with salt and pepper, then remove from heat and place on top of the hamburger patties. Serve with a fork.

Easiest Ever Stir Fry

What you will need:

1 bag Asian mixed vegetables

1 can water chestnuts

1 chicken breast

1 can Vienna sausage

½ cup soy sauce

Directions:

Cut the chicken into bite sized pieces, and add to a preheated skillet with 1 tablespoon olive oil. Cook slowly until the chicken is done, and set aside. Add the bag of veggies and the water chestnuts to the pan, and cook until completely cooked.

Add the chicken back into the pan, and pour the soy sauce over the top. Slice the can of Vienna sausages, and add to the stir fry. Cover the pan and turn down to low, then let sit for ten minutes, stirring occasionally.

Once all of the flavors have married, you can serve it. This is a bit of a larger recipe, and may serve up to 3.

Chapter 4 – Dinner Recipes

Let's face it, when it comes to dinner, no one knows what they want to do. It is the last meal of the day, and it tends to also be the biggest meal of the day. Dinners tend to go one of two ways.

Either (one) you are too tired to make something healthy and nice for your meal, or (two) you don't know what to make at this point because you have been working all day and don't have the mental energy to put into thinking out dinner.

Both of these situations are completely understandable, but they don't have to be that way. Here are some recipes that are not at all hard to make, but that you can whip up for dinner in a flash, and not have to worry about undoing the rest of your day.

Cheese and Broccoli Soup

What you will need:

2 cups broccoli florets

1 small onion

1 bag shredded sharp cheddar cheese

Salt and pepper

1 cup heavy cream

2 cups almond milk

Directions:

Pour the cream and milk into a pot on the stove, and turn onto medium high heat. As the cream is heating, chop the onion and broccoli as small as you can get them.

Add to the pot, and let simmer on the stove for 20 minutes. When the broccoli and onion are soft, slowly mix in the cheese, and stir until melted.

Using a stick blender, blend all ingredients until smooth, then season with salt and pepper, to taste. Let simmer for another 10 minutes, covered, then serve.

Note: If the soup is too thick (as it sometimes is with the cheese) you can add in a bit more of the almond milk. This will make it a lot thinner, and more manageable for younger people especially.

Cattle on a Bed

What you will need:

8 short ribs

2 large green leaf lettuce leaves

1 red onion

3 tablespoons BBQ sauce

3 tablespoons coconut milk

1 tomato

1 avocado

Directions:

Begin by mixing the barbeque sauce and the coconut milk in a small dish, and baste over the ribs. Slowly cook the ribs in the oven for one hour, on low, with the barbeque sauce.

Lay out the lettuce, and slice the onion and avocado. Arrange the onion and avocado pleasantly on the leaves, and chop the tomato as small as possible. Sprinkle the tomato on the leaves, and set aside.

When the ribs are done, separate them, 4 per plate, and arrange them nicely on each of the leaves of lettuce.

Serve immediately.

Note: this may be a bit dry, so you may need to add in a bit more coconut milk. Watch them casually in the oven, and if they seem to be getting dry, pull them out early, there are few things that are more disappointing than dry ribs on your lettuce!

Inside Out Burger

What you will need:

1 pound burger

2 slices bacon

2 slices cheddar cheese

1 small onion

1 tomato

2 leaves lettuce

Ketchup

Mayo

Salt and pepper, to taste

Directions:

Divide the hamburger into 4 sections, and flatten into 4 patties. Heat a skillet on the stove with a bit of olive oil, on medium high heat.

Slice the bacon into small bits, and chop the onion and tomato. Slice the cheese into thin strips as well.

Then, lay one of the patties on a plate, and pile half of each of these things on the patty.

Then, take the other patty, and lay it over the first patty. Carefully pinch the edges together, and place in the skillet.

Cook thoroughly, making sure the bacon is cooked on the inside as well.

Repeat the same steps for the other patty, then serve on the lettuce with mayo, ketchup, and salt and pepper.

Serve with a fork.

Meatball Boats

What you will need:

1 spaghetti squash

1 jar spaghetti sauce (garden vegetable)

1 bag shredded mozzarella cheese

1 small can mushrooms

½ pound hamburger

Directions:

Cook the spaghetti squash in the oven, covered in foil, at 350 degrees F for 1 hour. When it is done, set it aside to cool.

As it cools, divide the meat into 4 equal sized balls, and open the can of mushrooms.

Slice the spaghetti squash in half lengthwise.

Place the meatballs onto each half, and cover in spaghetti sauce.

Sprinkle the mushrooms on each boat, and generously cover with cheese.

Place back into the oven, and bake for another half an hour.

Once it is finished, slice the boats into strips, and serve immediately.

Creamy Chicken Delight

What you will need:

3 young green onions

2 chicken breasts

1 can cream of chicken soup

1 carton sour cream

½ package shredded cheddar cheese

Directions:

In 2 tablespoons olive oil, cook both chicken breasts on the stove in a skillet over medium high heat. As the chicken is cooking, chop the onion, leaving them in somewhat larger pieces.

In a baking dish, lay both chicken breasts, and set aside. Combine the soup and the sour cream, then mix in the green onion in the sour cream. Spread evenly over the chicken, and garnish with the shredded cheese.

Place in an oven preheated to 350 degrees F, and bake, covered for 15 minutes. Then, uncover the dish, and bake uncovered for an additional 5 minutes, or until the cheese has a nice, firm crust over the top of it.

Serve with a side salad of lettuce, almonds, and a nice vinaigrette.

Chapter 5 – Snacks and Desserts

It's no secret the favorite meal of the day is dessert. We bribe children with it, we work towards it ourselves, and it can even serve as a great reward to us for a job well done.

Don't skip out on dessert, and don't be afraid to let yourself indulge in this delectable meal. It is a mistake that a lot of people make, thinking they can't have dessert because of too many calories or mistakes like that.

Here are a few desserts that are perfect for any day of the week, not just Friday, and you will have something delightful to look forward to all day long.

Cheater Chocolate Sundae

What you will need:

Chocolate ice cream (Breyer's has come up with a whole new line of ice cream, one that is specifically designed for those who are on low carb diets. It is only 4 net grams of carbs per serving, and can be purchased at nearly any grocery store.)

Whipping cream

2 packets stevia

2 medium strawberries

1 cup crushed almonds

Directions:

Using an ice cream scoop, scoop two large ice cream balls into a dish. Repeat for the second dish. In a mixing bowl, combine the stevia and whipping cream, and mix with a blender until stiff.

Spoon the whipped cream on top of the ice cream, and place one strawberry per bowl. Garnish with the crushed almonds.

Note: This recipe calls for chocolate ice cream, but there are several different flavors that Breyer's has released, so you are really free to go with whatever you choose.

Guilt Free Chocolate Smoothie

What you will need:

2 cups chocolate almond milk

1 tablespoon cocoa powder

1 avocado

1 packet stevia

1 tablespoon peanut butter

½ cup whipped cream

Ice

Directions:

Place all ingredients besides the ice and whipped creaming into a blender, and blend on high until completely smooth. It can be difficult to get all of the powder mixed in, so you may need to turn the blender off, and scrape the powder down into the rest of the smoothie.

Add in the ice a few cubes at a time, and blend in. Add the ice cubes until the smoothie is the desired consistency, then divide into two separate glasses. Garnish the tops of the smoothies with whipped cream, and serve immediately.

Sprinkle Balls

What you will need:

1/4 cup peanut butter

½ cup chocolate chips

2 packets stevia

2 tablespoons almond flour

1 can sprinkles of your choice

Directions:

In a mixing bowl, combine the peanut butter, stevia, and almond flour. Stir until it is smooth. Melt the chocolate chips into a bowl, and pour into the peanut butter mix. Stir until it is completely mixed.

If it is too wet, add in more almond flour. You want it to be thick enough to form into balls. Once you can do that, you are ready to add in the sprinkles. Spread the sprinkles thickly on a plate, then roll the balls until they are covered in the sprinkles.

Place on a clean plate, and place in the freezer for an hour. Once they are chilled, you can enjoy them.

Snacks

While desserts are definitely the cup of tea of the day, we all greatly enjoy our snacks. It seems like there are endless hours stretching between meals, and it can be hard to make it from one meal to the next without a bit of a boost in between.

What makes these little power houses difficult, however, is the fact that few people plan on having snacks. They just go about their days until they realize they are hungry, then they hit the vending machine, or grab a bag of candy on their way through the store.

There is good news, however, and that is the fact you can make your own ketogenic snacks from scratch that will go perfectly with your eating plan, and help you get to where you want to be with your weight, your goals, and your life.

Of course, there is always the old standby of the handful of nuts, but that gets old and boring quickly. You want snacks that are going to be interesting, keep you satisfied, and best yet, keep you making them over and over again.

Sinking Boats

What you will need:

4 celery stalks

1 teaspoon garlic

Cream cheese

Almond pieces

Chocolate chips

Directions:

Wash and cut the celery stalks into smaller, more manageable sections, and fill with cream cheese. Sprinkle half of the stalks with garlic, and place pieces of almond in the cream cheese with the garlic.

In the pieces with no garlic, you can add the chocolate chips.

Dip and Dunks

What you will need:

¼ cup bleu cheese

½ cup plain yogurt

2 packets stevia

2 cucumbers

2 stalks celery

Directions:

Wash the cucumbers and the celery, and slice them into small spears. Next, in a small dish, mix the bleu cheese, yogurt, and stevia. Blend until smooth, breaking up the larger pieces of cheese if necessary.

Dip the cucumber and celery in the dip, or whatever else you think sounds good, you really can't go wrong with this delightful addition to your day!

American Flag Delight

What you will need:

1 large strawberry

¼ cup blueberries

1 carton cottage cheese (full fat)

Directions:

Slice the strawberry into small spears. Then, take ½ of the tub of cottage cheese and mix with the blueberries and strawberries. Take care not to overmix, as you want the colors to swirl into a delight of red, white, and blue.

Once it is mixed, you can serve. It is ready to go right off a spoon!

Remember to mix and match as you please.

These recipes are all perfect for your ketogenic eating plan. There are very few carbs in any of these recipes, and they are all perfect if you want to eat each one for breakfast, lunch, and dinner all in the same day.

You need to keep in mind that there are carbs in pretty near everything that you eat, and the goal of this diet is not to be carb free, but to cut down on carbs as much as possible, while getting the high fat content.

This is why you don't want to get anything that is low on fat, and go for the full amount of all of it. If you are ever in doubt with any of the fruits, feel free to cut the amount in the recipe, or replace them with something else.

The key to the success of this diet is to make it work for you. Sure, you are going to have to follow some guidelines and rules if you want to be successful, but overall you really do have a lot of say on what you are making.

Once you know how to follow the limit you can have of carbs in a day, there isn't

anything that will stop you. You can eat out, eat at anyone's house, or just grab a quick bite, while staying well within your limit.

This is more than just a diet, it is a real lifestyle that you are a part of. You can make it happen, and you will see the results in your body, in a remarkably short amount of time.

Find what you like, and make the things that you want. You can read the labels and figure out just how many carbs you are eating, and you can adjust what you are eating day to day to make sure you are under your limit.

Either way, I know that these recipes are going to be perfect for you and your newly found lifestyle, and in a matter of days you are going to see a drastic difference in your waist line, in how your clothes fit, and how you are feeling.

Your confidence will soar, and it will be like you are experiencing a whole new life. Now get out there and embrace it with everything you've got!

Conclusion

There you have it, 20 delicious and easy to make recipes that will fit into any family's budget, and fit the bill of even the pickiest eater. You can say goodbye to the days of stressing about what you can and can't eat, and how you are going to lose those annoying pounds that just seem to want to hang on.

These recipes are your key to success, and you will love the results you will see as soon as you start this diet. There is a life out there just waiting for you to jump in and take your part in it, so what are you waiting for?

Get out there and show the world what you are made of.